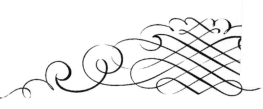

ISBN 978-1-330-04182-6
PIBN 10011198

This book is a reproduction of an important historical work. Forgotten Books uses
state-of-the-art technology to digitally reconstruct the work, preserving the original format
whilst repairing imperfections present in the aged copy. In rare cases, an imperfection in
the original, such as a blemish or missing page, may be replicated in our edition. We do,
however, repair the vast majority of imperfections successfully; any imperfections that
remain are intentionally left to preserve the state of such historical works.

1 MONTH OF
FREE
READING

at
www.ForgottenBooks.com

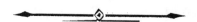

By purchasing this book you are eligible for one month membership to ForgottenBooks.com, giving you unlimited access to our entire collection of over 1,000,000 titles via our web site and mobile apps.

To claim your free month visit:

www.forgottenbooks.com/free11198

English
Français
Deutsche
Italiano
Español
Português

www.forgottenbooks.com

Mythology Photography **Fiction**
Fishing Christianity **Art** Cooking
Essays Buddhism Freemasonry
Medicine **Biology** Music **Ancient
Egypt** Evolution Carpentry Physics
Dance Geology **Mathematics** Fitness
Shakespeare **Folklore** Yoga Marketing
Confidence Immortality Biographies
Poetry **Psychology** Witchcraft
Electronics Chemistry History **Law**
Accounting **Philosophy** Anthropology
Alchemy Drama Quantum Mechanics
Atheism Sexual Health **Ancient History**
Entrepreneurship Languages Sport
Paleontology Needlework Islam
Metaphysics Investment Archaeology
Parenting Statistics Criminology
Motivational

Prize Essay.

EVILS OF TOBACCO,

AS THEY AFFECT

Body, Mind, and Morals.

BY

REV. DWIGHT BALDWIN.

"Abstain from all appearance of evil."—PAUL.

NEW YORK:

FOWLERS AND WELLS, PUBLISHERS,

CLINTON HALL, 131 NASSAU STREET.

LONDON: 142 Strand.

BOSTON:
No. 142 Washington St.

1854.

PHILADELPHIA:
No. 231 Arch Street.

1854.

(76. 72. 1843.)

Prize Essay.

EVILS OF TOBACCO,

AS THEY AFFECT

BODY, MIND, AND MORALS.

BY REV. DWIGHT BALDWIN.

"Abstain from all appearance of evil."—PAUL.

Fowlers and Wells, Publishers, Clinton Hall, 131 Nassau street, New York.

To this Essay was awarded one of the prizes offered in April, 1853, through the "Water-Cure Journal" and the "American Phrenological Journal," by a benevolent and philanthropic gentleman of the State of New York, who prefers for the present to remain unknown, but who hopes, by its publication, to aid in suppressing a degrading and dangerous habit, and in preventing the young from ignorantly becoming its willing victims.

The series of Tobacco Essays of which this Tract forms a part, is but the beginning of the end of what he designs. Should the world be found to have been improved by his efforts, he will consider it an ample reward for all he has done, or may do hereafter. Who will aid him by circulating this Tract?

ALL the lower orders of the animal creation obey the instincts of their nature. Man alone, as Dr. Mussey observes, " seeks to poison or destroy his instincts, to turn topsy-turvy the laws of his being, and to make himself as unlike as possible to that which he was obviously designed to be."

This is eminently true in regard to what men allow themselves to eat and drink. The fact that millions of our race form artificial appetites, and gratify those appetites at the expense of health and life, cannot be questioned.

The use of Tobacco, though often the subject of jest and trifling, is, nevertheless, one of vast importance; for it deeply affects the interests of thousands and millions of our race. Confined for nearly 5,600 years, so far as we know, to Central America, and some parts of the West Indies, it is wonderful that, in less than three centuries, it has spread over the whole world. It has found its way, despite the edicts of kings, into every nation, and monarchs and no- bles, as well as peasants, have come under its dominion. No plant has been so widely diffused ; none has had more infatuated devotees ; and if we except the sugar-cane and the vine, none has exerted more influence upon the bodies, minds, and characters of mankind. It becomes all, therefore, to inquire whether this influence is salutary or hurtful.

In treating of this subject, I propose to indicate, 1. The medicinal proper- ties of Tobacco. 2. Some of the common and necessary effects of Tobacco on its habitual consumers. 3. To mention briefly the diseases it occasions,

(1)

4. To examine the excuses made for its use. 5. To offer some other considerations which should dissuade men from using Tobacco. 6. To indicate the methods of promoting a cure of the Tobacco habit.

I. MEDICINAL PROPERTIES.

What are the medicinal powers of Tobacco? This question is easily answered, as none of its properties are obscure. On every system not accustomed to its use, they declare themselves " as the sin of Sodom." Neither has there ever been any dispute among medical men, as to what those medicinal properties are. Whatever medical authority we open, we find that Tobacco has certain diuretic powers attributed to it; that it is an emetic of great energy; that, in certain circumstances, it acts as a cathartic; but that its most prominent and powerful quality is the *narcotic*. The general effect of *narcotics* is to allay excitement and nervous irritation, to quiet restlessness, to diminish sensibility, relieve pain, and promote sleep. These effects are produced only by small doses. In excessive doses, their effects are stupor, convulsions, prostration, and death. Of all narcotics known, not more than one can vie with Tobacco for deadly power, when used under circumstances which favor its action.*

Dr. Chapman, of Philadelphia, has described Tobacco under the head of emetics; though he remarks that " it has other properties, which give it as strong a claim to a different location in the *materia medica.*" He is perfectly right in this arrangement. Even the nauseousness alone of Tobacco would give it a place among emetics. But Tobacco has higher claims to the office of an emetic than merely its power on the olfactories. Its power of disturbing any stomach which is in its natural state, is inherent and energetic. Not long since, a child, in Massachusetts, sent to a store, was persuaded by the clerk to swallow a little Tobacco, which he denominated good. Who could think there was any harm in an article of such common use? But it brought on such a fearful vomiting as no power of the physician could stay. A mortal paleness, convulsions and death soon followed. The silly clerk was guilty of manslaughter. Unlike all other emetics, this seems equally powerful

---

* Medical writers always make a distinction between narcotics and stimulants. By narcotics they mean medicines which diminish action and stupefy the body and mind; by stimulants, those which increase the action of the system. But no definite line can ever be drawn between these two classes of medicines, they run so insensibly into each other. All the narcotics, especially in moderate doses, produce a temporary excitement of the vital powers, and this is followed by a far greater depression. On the other hand, the increased action produced by stimulants is followed by a depression of bodily and mental powers, similar to that which succeeds the use of narcotics. This depression is always at least equal to, and generally far greater than, the previous excitement. Indeed, the alcoholic liquors, and other stimulants, taken in large or dangerous doses, produce a prostration of all the vital powers, and death, without any previous excitement, just like the most potent narcotics. Opium and Tobacco, famous narcotics, are as decidedly intoxicating as are rum, brandy, or any of the tribe of drunkard-makers.

whether taken internally, or applied externally to the body. A cataplasm of Tobacco-leaves, applied to the chest, over the region of the stomach, has caused alarming symptoms of retching and vomiting, which have not ceased, even when the cause has been removed ; and we have read of hireling soldiers who have brought upon themselves vomiting and convulsions by wearing Tobacco-leaves under their arm-pits, that they might be excused from duty.

With such various and manifest medicinal powers, one would suppose that Tobacco would be a valuable article in the *materia medica*. But the contrary is the fact. It is seldom used by physicians in any part of the world, and never, perhaps, except in extreme cases. With the whole tribe of Tobacco consumers, it is entirely useless as a remedy in disease ; and, with all others, it is extremely uncertain in its operation. The greatest objection, however, to its use is, that it so frequently takes on the most furious and deadly action, utterly beyond all control, so that the remedy becomes more formidable than almost any disease.

Tobacco should not be called a remedy ; for there cannot be a doubt that it causes ten thousand cases of disease where it cures one. It is universally reckoned among the poisons, and with as much reason as is the fang of the rattlesnake or the viper. Let us hear what the doctors say.

Dr. Cox, of Brooklyn, a Doctor of Divinity, says : " The dirty weed is poisonous and offensive, contrary to nature, and at war with it." John Quincy Adams, a Doctor of Laws, speaks from experience of the " pernicious operation of Tobacco on the stomach and the nerves." Dr. Paris, of London, says : " Tobacco is endued with energetic poisonous properties, producing generally a universal tremor, which is rarely the result of other poisons." The United States Dispensatory, compiled by medical professors of Philadelphia, says : " There are two poisonous principles in Tobacco ; the one, called *Nicotia*, or *Nicotin*, is of an alkaline nature, and in its action on the animal system, is one of the most virulent poisons known. A single drop of it in a state of concentrated solution, was sufficient to destroy the life of a dog ; and small birds perished at the approach of a tube containing it. Tobacco also affords, by distillation, an empyreumatic oil, which is a most virulent poison. One drop applied to the tongue, or injected into the rectum, of a cat, occasions death in about five minutes ; and double the quantity, administered in the same manner to a dog, was followed by the same result. This oil is of a dark brown color, and smells exactly like Tobacco-pipes which have been long used." I may add also, on the authority of Dr. Paris, that every smoker, by the action of fire on Tobacco, constantly manufactures this oil, and experiments with it, not on cats, but on the most delicate and vital organs of his own body. Dr. Franklin discovered this oil by passing Tobacco-smoke through water. The oily matter which floated on the surface of the water was applied to the tongue of a cat, and destroyed life in a few minutes. Dr. Mussey tried many similar experiments on cats, dogs, and other animals, to show the poisonous power of the oil of Tobacco.

There is no necessity for multiplying authorities on this point; but it will not be amiss just to refer to Orfila, a well-known writer on poisons. He divides all poisons into four classes:

1. *Irritating poisons*, such as occasion inflammation, and more or less dissolution of the parts they touch; such as *arsenic*, and most mineral poisons.

2. *Narcotic or stupefying poisons*, such as opium, henbane, prussic acid, &c.

3. *Acrid narcotic poisons*, in which he includes poison-mushrooms, the nux-vomica or strychnine, the Bohon Upas of Java, Tobacco, poison-hemlock, belladonna, or deadly nightshade, &c.

4. *The septic or putrefying poisons*, as the venom of the viper, asp, copper-head, rattlesnake, scorpion, &c.

Such is the rank assigned by a great physician to the famous weed we have under consideration. If we now refer to the arrangement of the botanist, we find Tobacco in the natural order *Solanaceæ*, which is famed for poisons. In the artificial arrangement of Linnæus, it is found in Class 5th, Order 1st; of the whole of which order, the botanist says. the degree of their poison is in proportion to the paleness of their color and the nauseousness of their smell.

II. EFFECTS.

Let us now speak of some of the common and necessary effects of Tobacco on its habitual consumers. After all that has been said of the poisonous and powerful qualities of Tobacco, we shall not be slow to conclude that the influence of such an article on the human system cannot be a matter of indifference. We must admit that it is a foe to the health and comfort of man, of no ordinary power. Mr. Lane, a writer on this subject who had much experience in Tobacco-using, says:

"If the habitual use of Tobacco did not produce the most fearful results, it would be a mystery in the philosophy of causes and their effects. And yet, to show the deleterious effects of Tobacco on the human constitution, so as to convince all, and especially so as to convince the consumers of Tobacco, is not always an easy task. The difficulty arises, first, from the fact that, after the first loathing of Tobacco is past, its influence is slow and insidious; never violent, rapid, and inflammatory, like the effects of ardent spirit. With all the manifestly ruinous power of alcoholic drinks on health, reputation, and fortunes, yet multitudes can never be convinced that they are necessarily hurtful. Millions hold to their *prudent use.* How much more difficult, then, must it be to convince men that there is any danger in the gentle, soothing powers of this loved narcotic! Fashion too unites with appetite in throwing a kind of spell over the Tobacco-consumer, which, however absurd and wicked the habit may appear to some, yet binds its victims in iron fetters. Arguments used to such, too often seem as powerless as they would in breaking up the spell of a rattlesnake."

There is on earth no such inveterate trio as opium, rum, and Tobacco; no other articles have held such sway over the appetites of men ; none have so bewitched and chained them ; none wasted so much time and money, or spread so much mischief over the world. Opium has reigned only over a few nations and a few individuals of all nations. Millions are already alarmed at rum's doings, and the Maine Law is on its way round the world ; but only a few are doing serious battle against the weed. Their number is increasing ; but when we see what throngs, from kings, nobles, scholars, and all classes of enlightened lands, down to the naked, squalid savages of heathen nations, pamper their animal appetites with these nauseous fumes and nauseous tastes, we may well ask, Where will the dominion of Tobacco end? It is this bewitching power of appetite, this subordination of the soul and reason of man to the beastly part of his nature, that makes arguments against this trio of curses so powerless. Still the opposer of Tobacco should go on, trusting that reason and facts will yet demonstrate the absurdity of men's using habitually such a potent drug ; that so large a portion of our race is not always to be narcotized ; and that sense will yet be subordinated, and the weed return to its original owner—the Tobacco-worm.

1. The first effect I shall mention, produced in the system by the continual use of Tobacco, is creating an appetite for the repetition of the indulgence. Almost all articles of diet employed by men, when long used, cloy the appetite, and a change is desired. This is especially true of animal food. The richest viands soonest satiate, and desire is changed to aversion. For articles of vegetable food, in daily use all our lives, no such appetite is ever formed as for such stimulants and narcotics as alcohol, opium, and Tobacco. Even bread, the staff of life, can be dispensed with, and not leave any great or painful feeling of vacuity behind. These are the general laws in relation to all articles which contribute to the growth and nourishment of the human body. Alcohol, opium, and Tobacco, are always notorious exceptions to these laws. They never cloy the appetite. The users of them are never satiated by frequent or long-continued indulgence. On the contrary, as daily observation shows, the longer the habit of using these articles is continued, the more inveterate does the desire for them become, till the article used becomes part and parcel of the man's existence, without which there is no rest or comfort for him. The appetites for these three articles are all formed on the same general principles ; they depend on the same laws of the animal economy ; and that of the chewer or smoker for his favorite article, does not yield in strength and inveteracy to either of its compeers. An appetite, it may be called at first, but it soon becomes a longing, hankering, torturing desire for the object, which increases more and more in intensity, the longer the habit is continued, till it forms an absolute and imperious passion, demanding almost constant gratification, and which must be gratified at all hazards. I should not have mentioned the appetite formed for Tobacco among the effects it produces on the system, had I not supposed that the strength of the appetite would show pretty exactly how far the system was

perverted from its natural state, and, of course, how much injury the article was doing to the man. The fact of such an appetite being formed, is all I have dwelt on here ; the nature of the appetite will appear more clearly when we consider,

2. The manner in which Tobacco operates on the system ; which is always by exciting the nervous powers of the body. The same is true of opium and alcohol. Alcohol excites the nerves, and inflames every part with which it comes in contact. Opium is a more powerful exciter than Tobacco, and being quickly followed by its depressing or narcotic effect, is valuable as an anodyne. Tobacco is more gentle in its exciting powers, but possesses more, by far, of the deadly narcotic energy. All these articles excite the the system above its ordinary or healthful tone, which exaltation is speedily followed, as a matter of course, by an exhaustion and a sinking or depression of all the bodily and mental powers. The universal law, well known to all who study the human system, is, that the exhaustion and depression of the system caused by stimulants is proportioned to the height to which it has been raised above the healthy tone ; but in the case of the purer narcotics, such as Tobacco, the excitement is more moderate, and passes off quickly, and the depression and stupidity bear a much greater proportion than in case of stimulants. Indeed, in regard to Tobacco, probably the habitual user knows very little of its exciting qualities. The soothing soporific or stupefying powers of the article are those of which he is sensible. When Tobacco first begins to exert its exciting or soothing effect on the smoker or chewer, he may feel something of the sensual enjoyment which belongs to the drunkard during the incipient stages of intoxication. But he soon reaches a point where bodily comfort ends, and where a sense of exhaustion or vacuity comes over him. No matter by what name we call it, there is a sinking, flagging, typhoid state of all the powers of body and mind. Every Tobacco-user feels this sense of want to a greater or less degree. Nature has experienced a temporary depression, and is in distress. Relief can only be found in a repetition of his accustomed stimulus. So long as nothing but unstimulating. nutritive articles of diet enter the body, all its functions are left to go on in a uniform tone of action, and the result would naturally be a healthful tone of all parts of the system. It needs no process of reasoning to show that a man, in such a state of the bodily functions, possesses the highest animal enjoyment which can be uniformly maintained in the human system. But wherever there is a violation of nature's established laws, in the application to the body of agents which nature never designed for such application, there must always be a penalty—sometimes immediate, but much oftener delayed and multiplied into a series of penalties reaching through successive years.

It is not to be understood that the evil effects of Tobacco will always appear after a moderate transgression, or for a very limited period. There is in the system a wonderful power of accommodating itself to noxious matters, and often a vigorous constitution will resist their influence for many years

There is no doubt but that many, especially the strong and muscular, have made a careful use of Tobacco all their lives, and its evil effects have not been very apparent. But what is maintained is, that there is always in it a tendency to produce these evil effects, and no man should take it for granted that his system is proof against its power. The continued application every day, perhaps every hour, for successive years, of so powerful a drug as Tobacco to the delicate organs of the human system, especially where the appetite is increasing, and the system learning to depend more and more on the artificial stimulus, will inevitably wear upon the nervous power—the life of the body. The nerves will become enfeebled and deranged to a greater or less extent, the vigor of the stomach will give way, other functions of the body will depart more or less from their natural state, involving a consequent sacrifice of the comfort of body and mind. The victim of these habits seeks to restore the loss by applying more and more frequently the cause of all his trouble. He strengthens and soothes his aching, agitated nerves by that which has induced all their weakness and agitation, and which will continue to aggravate all these evils in time to come. To quench the fire which has begun to burn him, he, like the drunkard, adds more fuel.

Reformed chewers and smokers, who have been long victims of the weed, have described the evils which it inflicts on the body and mind, with an eloquence which ought long since to have gone to the heart of every Tobacco-consumer in the world. Mr. Lane, who speaks from abundant experience, says : " It causes a thousand disagreeable and painful feelings which the poor victim knows not to be the necessary results of his pernicious indulgence. In mind and body he is miserable ; if asked to describe his feelings, he can only say, like the man possessed among the tombs, *their name is legion.* To find relief, he chews his cud, or sucks his pipe, or suffocates himself with Tobacco-dust ; but instead of light, behold, darkness and the shadow of death come upon him."

A sea-captain, of more than ordinary good sense, was lately asked why he had left off smoking Tobacco. He replied, "I had two reasons for it; first, I found that when I smoked, I had no appetite for food ; I could eat nothing with comfort. But what alarmed me most was, that when I went to bed without a cigar, a kind of horrors came over me. I felt dreadfully, and could not go to sleep. I would get up and take a cigar, and then have a quiet night's rest. I thought," he added, "if I was so dependent on a foreign stimulant for comfort, it was high time to leave it off. I quit smoking—my appetite returned, is always good—and I can now go to sleep at night more quietly without a cigar, than I could formerly with one." The horrors of which the captain spoke, are nothing more nor less than the sufferings of the body and mind from exhaustion and derangement of the nervous system. The same evil, carried to a greater extent, would produce *delirium tremens,* of which medical writers have recorded cases, as caused by an excessive use of Tobacco.

After these remarks and the examples which have been cited, we shall not be at a loss in regard to what causes the appetite for alcohol, opium, or Tobacco : such an appetite as is never formed for any article of food with which we are acquainted. It is an appetite which is located, not in the mouth, nor in the palate, nor in the throat, nor yet in the stomach. Doubtless the palate and stomach would of themselves always continue to loathe all these articles ; certainly they would never cease to revolt at the nauseous taste of Tobacco. But a real disease has been created in the whole body, even to the extremities of countless nerves which branch over it, by applying to them excitants of a higher tone than are consistent with a state of health. The longer a man sustains his system by these artificial stimulants, the greater will the sinking be which follows the use of them ; the greater the nervous debility and nervous suffering. Tobacco, no less than rum or opium, leaves behind it a longing, voracious, aching void, which all the food in the world cannot fill. The torment of the chewer or smoker, when the cud or the pipe is withheld beyond the customary interval, is not imaginary ; it is real. The sense of want may be referred by the individual to the stomach, or to some other organ ; but it is the whole system, body and mind, which is in distress and cries out for help. The amount of that distress is precisely the amount of appetite which the man has acquired for Tobacco ; so that we hazard nothing when we say, that the strength of a man's appetite for Tobacco, in whatever way used, will tell him, with almost mathematical precision, the mischief it has already done to his body ; and how great is the necessity of his abandoning, at once, chewing and smoking, if he would prolong his days, or consult his real comfort.

We cannot sufficiently wonder at the folly of thousands, perhaps millions, who chew or smoke Tobacco, thinking it adds to their animal enjoyment. That savage nations should seek enjoyment in this way is not wonderful. But all the civilized world ought to know, that the highest and most permanent corporeal enjoyment belongs only to man in perfect health. When every organ of the body is in healthful play, doing well and uniformly the work assigned to it in the system ; neither excited above the tone of nature, depressed below it, nor disturbed by noxious powers ; when the mind is active, the spirit buoyant, the food sweet, and exercise and labor equally delightful, who does not know that all the drugs in the world would no more heighten the enjoyment of such a man, than they would that of skipping lambs or gambolling children? You can no more improve Nature's established and happy medium of action in the body, than you can the water which God pours out of the clouds, by mingling it with brandy or arsenic. For every ounce of pleasure we extort from the body by artificial means, we shall doubtless always pay in pounds of pain.

III. DISEASES.

Let us now refer to some of the diseases, or rather classes of disease, caused by the use of Tobacco.

1. As Tobacco exhausts and deranges the nervous powers, it is evident that its consumers must be more liable than others to many, and perhaps to the whole train, of nervous diseases, which inflict upon our race a frightful proportion of the miseries which fall to the lot of man in this world. Judging from the published experience of numerous chewers and smokers, we must conclude that few of all the consumers of Tobacco are allowed wholly to escape the torments of this class of diseases.

2. Tobacco is peculiarly calculated to produce diseases to which the stomach is liable; and especially those forms which go under the name of *dyspepsia*, with all their kindred train of evils. This is just what we ought to expect from the use of such a poison. In the action of chewing and smoking, some of the strength of Tobacco will find its way directly into the stomach. Chewing especially wastes a portion of the saliva which is absolutely essential to the work of digestion; and both chewing and smoking poison the portion which is allowed to flow into the stomach, and which ought to go there pure as nature has formed it. There is still a third method by which Tobacco promotes dyspepsia in its votaries, which is, through its general action on the system. The nerves of the stomach are among the most delicate and sensitive in the body, and it is mainly through them that Tobacco inflicts evils on other parts of the system. While, therefore, it wastes and deranges the nervous powers of the whole system, those of the stomach not only share in the mischief, but often receive the heaviest infliction.

After the stomach has been for a long time subjected to the potent energies of Tobacco, is it strange that it should become insensible to the stimulus of common food; that the power of digestion should be diminished, or even destroyed? The testimony of physicians is confirmed by the experience of chewers and smokers, that Tobacco diminishes the appetite; and that when forsaken, appetite returns, and the weight of the body is increased. We seldom listen to the history of a reformed Tobacco-consumer, without feeling that he has become acquainted with some of dyspepsia's bluest horrors.

3. I have only room to mention one other class of diseases produced by Tobacco, and that is, diseases of the mind, or those in which the mind is greatly affected. Such is the intimate connection between the nerves and the mind, that it is impossible that one should be affected without affecting the other. The nerves are all branches of the brain; the brain is the seat of the mind, and it is only through the medium of the nerves that the mind holds intercourse with the external world. All have heard of the ruinous effects of opium on the mind; of the mental imbecility and the uncontrollable irritability of temper produced by the habitual use of this drug, through its action upon the nerves. Tobacco is more slow and insidious in its operation, and its effects on the system are, therefore, sometimes overlooked, or ascribed to other causes; but we have abundant reason to think that it is no less sure or baleful in its effects on the body and on the mind,

A writer of long experience in the use of Tobacco says : "The disastrous influence of Tobacco upon the mind is no less fearful than upon the body. No tongue or pen can describe the intellectual ruin occasioned by it." Another enumerates, among the effects of Tobacco, enfeebling the memory, a confusion of ideas, irritability of temper, want of energy and steadiness of purpose, melancholy, fatuity, and insanity. Prof. Mussey has given a fearful list of diseases which may arise from the use of Tobacco ; but perhaps it is not necessary to enumerate particular diseases. If we have proof that the influence of Tobacco is detrimental to the nervous system, the grand medium of the life of the body, and to the stomach, the grand centre of support and growth to all parts of the system, we may safely take it for granted that Tobacco will pave the way for almost every disease to which human nature is liable.

IV. EXCUSES

1. Some think they have found a relief for phthisical or asthmatic symptoms in Tobacco-smoke. It is possible that Tobacco, by its emetic or narcotic power, may have relieved asthma. But, on the other hand, we have known of asthma's being cured by forsaking Tobacco, which had been used habitually ; and we have the highest medical authority for believing that consumption and bleeding at the lungs have been caused by the habitual use of Tobacco. Whatever relief an occasional dose of Tobacco may afford, it soon becomes no medicine to the habitual user of it.

2. Many believe that Tobacco is necessary to aid the work of digestion. By its exciting and soothing effect, it may have made the stomach more easy under a single meal. But it is equally true, that the meal which required foreign aid for its digestion, should never have been taken. It is not in the nature of Tobacco to give permanent aid in the work of digestion. It may destroy the power of the stomach, but never increase it. Dr. Mussey, than whom we have no higher authority, says, "The opinion that Tobacco is necessary to promote digestion, is altogether erroneous."

Pres. Hitchcock, who wrote on Dyspepsia, says: "The common opinion, that Tobacco, in some of its forms, is serviceable for headaches, weak eyes, purifying the breath, cold and watery stomachs, &c., is a mere delusion."

3. Some smoke Tobacco to prevent obesity. Instead of taking a medicine, it might be well for such to live in an unhealthy climate, which would effectually keep down the tone of health.

4. Probably the largest number who would offer any one excuse for using Tobacco, would plead its necessity as a preservative of the teeth. A multitude of salutary qualities were ascribed, in former times, to this vile weed, as well as to that greatest of all curses, ardent spirit—and, among others, the power of preventing decay in the teeth. Dr. Mussey says : "The notion that the use of Tobacco preserves the teeth, is supported neither by physiology nor by observation," and that it would rather accelerate than

retard their decay. Another worthy medical professor remarks: "It is impossible that an article which does so much to injure the powers of the stomach as does Tobacco, should not also, sooner or later, injure the teeth." Doubtless there are many preservatives of the teeth, far superior to Tobacco.

With all the pleas before us which have ever been made for chewing or smoking, we may conclude, that the cases are rare in which man could derive help from Tobacco which he could not better find in some other article; and that probably no man of our race ever yet had a valid excuse for the habitual use of so powerful and poisonous a drug. The habitual use of Tobacco was never calculated to promote health or substantial comfort, or to prolong life. It destroys all these. Notwithstanding the slow and insidious manner in which it poisons the vitals and undermines the constitution, it is yet seen that it occasions, everywhere, a frightful waste of life. In the United States, intelligent physicians have estimated that 20,000 die every year, from the use of Tobacco; and in Germany, where the streets, as well as the houses, are literally befogged with Tobacco-smoke, the physicians have calculated that, of all the deaths which occur between the ages of eighteen and thirty-five, *one-half* originate in the waste of the constitution by smoking! Such opinions as these, from the men who ought to know, should startle all the world, and bring chewers and smokers to their senses, in regard to the powers of this Indian weed, and the effect of habits which too many have been inclined, hitherto, to call harmless.

V. DISSUASIVES.

1. The first is a consideration which has weight, or ought to have, with all men, in this world of many wants. It is the *expense* of using Tobacco. If Tobacco is *useful* or *necessary* to health, we need not be scrupulous as to the amount we expend upon it. If it were simply for the gratification of an animal appetite, without adding to or detracting from the sum of our health or happiness, to lay out expense on such an article would seem to us all, at best, *a childish folly*. But if it can be shown to be positively *hurtful*, prejudicial to the vital functions, endangering health and shortening life, then to expend money on it is worse than folly—it is *madness*, and should be classed with what is expended on the cups of the drunkard—an expense to which he is impelled by a depraved appetite, while he knows it is hurrying himself to ruin, and preparing beggary for his children. We are all stewards of possessions, greater or less, which God has intrusted to our care, and which we are allowed to use for our own good and the good of others; but never have we the right to use a farthing to our own hurt, any more than we have for the injury of our fellow-men.

The young are apt to make very little account of small sums which they expend for their own gratification, or to comply with the fashions of the day.

But in what is expended on Tobacco, they should remember that there is likely to be a daily and constant demand upon them, which, in course of years, must necessarily swell to a considerable sum. Some expend but little at the outset ; but the appetite once formed, no one knows to what extent it will carry him. It is a very moderate cigar-smoker who spends only 6 cents a day ; and yet it amounts to $21.90 a year ; a sum which would be called an enormous tax, if laid on a young man for the purposes of government, or for the support of religious institutions. The same trifling sum, if put to annual interest, would, in thirty years, amount to $3,529 30 ; and who does not wish that cigars were banished from the world, when he thinks in how many hundred ways this sum might have contributed to the real comfort and improvement of a man in moderate circumstances ; or how much good it might have done, if laid out in educating and elevating his children? Or what man would not like such a sum to leave as a legacy to his children, instead of leaving to them his own miserable, filthy, Tobacco-habit?—a habit kept, perhaps, by the father within moderate bounds, but often, in the son, running beyond all bounds, without regard to expense.

But how many thousands on thousands are there in the land, who spend on cigars 12½ cents a day, $45 a year, or more than $7,000 in thirty years! This is the sum which every free negro in Cuba is said to spend on this degrading luxury ; which alone is sufficient to bind that class down to ignorance and degradation, in all future time. Many too there are among us, not rich, who devote 25 cents daily to cigars ; and some are miserable if they do not have 50 cents' worth to soothe their aching and distracted nerves. Let us remember, too, that this amazing Tobacco taxation does not fall mainly on the rich ; it falls equally on the middling and lower orders of society ; on multitudes of hard-working men, who have to struggle with privation and poverty ; who cannot afford their children the facilities of schools and academies, in this day of education ; who cannot purchase even a moiety of the rich literature with which genius is filling every enlightened land ; it falls on the hardy soldier, and on the wandering sailor who puffs his way over the ocean. It falls heavily too on students in every department of learning. "The cigar bill," we are told, "of many a student, clerk, and stripling, exceeds his board bill. The students of some of our colleges are estimated to pay annually from $6000 to $8000 for this vile luxury." It should be added, too, that Tobacco is the great generator of idle habits in the world, and what is lost by idleness is always estimated higher than the money expended.

If we now turn to the expense of smoking in some communities, we shall be astonished at our statistics, and wish to call in question the operations of arithmetic. The consumption of cigars alone, in the city of New-York, in 1851, was computed at $10,000 a day ; while the whole city paid but $8,500 a day for bread ; this would be $3,650,000 a year, for cigars alone. The Grand Erie Canal, three hundred and sixty-four miles long, the longest in the world, with its eighteen aqueducts and eighty-four locks, was made in six years, and cost over $7,000,000. The cigar bill of New York city would have paid the whole in two years. If a line of Atlantic steamers, the pride of the ocean, were all sunk, how soon would the cigar-money of that one city rebuild the whole! The annual cost of Tobacco in the whole United States is computed at $30,000,000. This sum would scarcely cover the labor of one and a half million men who are engaged in the cultivation of it; nor would it include all the idle hours and days of Tobacco-consumers. Is there a benevolent man in the world whose heart will not be pained at the thought of such immense wealth expended on an unnatural, artificial, and absurd appetite—an appetite which forty-nine in fifty of Tobacco-victims themselves will own had better never have been formed; an appetite which can do nothing less than injure, to some extent, all who use it; and which on some falls with a blighting power, unnerving the body and stultifying the mind!

Tobacco broods like an incubus over every chewer and smoker; it is a curse to the whole nation just in proportion as it is used. With the single exception of intoxicating drinks, what is there which would do more to change and deteriorate a nation's character than the universal use of Tobacco?

If the Tobacco consumption in the United States goes on in future, increasing as it has for twenty years past, have we not reason to fear that the nation of active, inventive, enterprising, efficient Yankees, flying all over the world, will be actually smoked down into a nation as phlegmatic and stationary as the smoking Dutchmen of Holland?

2. Another consideration to be remembered is, that whatever are the evils of Tobacco, to the individual or to the community, they will go on augmenting as long as the evil remains. The few keep such an evil habit within narrow bounds; the multitude go as appetite leads the way, just like the votaries of ardent spirits.

3. Another dissuasive from the use of Tobacco is the filthy character of the habit. We need only to name this topic to have it understood, as there are but few who have not, at times, been more or less annoyed by the offensiveness of those who use Tobacco. There are no laws more universally established, in refined society, than those which demand cleanliness of person and cleanly habits in all the intercourse of men with each other; and which proscribe all offensive or disgusting practices, as suited only to savage and barbarous nations, or to some of the lower orders of animals. The rules of refined society on such matters, and genuine politeness, are always one and the same thing. The three practices of chewing, smoking, and snuffing, are violations of all rules of cleanliness. It is not clear which is the greatest violation. We seldom or never hear even the victims of these habits defending them against the charge of being offensive and disgusting; and yet, strange to tell, they are not only tolerated among men who belong to the highest orders of society, but among thousands of such, especially the young,

they have grown into such a bewitching fashion, that one is ashamed to be seen among his companions unless his mouth is armed with a cud, or his head enveloped in Tobacco-fumes. Some carry these filthy practices into all the society they frequent, endangering all who do not keep at a distance, or to the windward; endangering all that female ingenuity has devised to make home pleasant, or poisoning the air that all are compelled to breathe. Others there are, better educated, more refined in manners, who never forget that their habits are utterly inconsistent with the rules of good society, who drop the cud or cigar at the door they enter, and who willingly take the "smoking-car," or the smoking end of the steamboat. But even such seem to forget that it is easier to part with the cigar than it is with the fetid breath it has occasioned, which often affects others, even to vomiting. They cannot know how nauseous the weed is to others, when it has become so delightful to them. That such unnatural and offensive habits should ever have found a place outside of the precincts of savage life, is a wonder. It is a greater wonder that men who claim to rank with the refined should allow any thing in their habits which is to unfit them for society; and that, when they find themselves severed off, like lepers of old, shame does not kindle into indignation, and indignation lead to reformation; but the greatest wonder of all is, that the fair sex, who take the lead in all that is refined and lovely, in enlightened lands; married ladies, who have a deep interest in the habits of husbands and sons, have not, long since, brought all the power of their persuasive influence to bear upon these habits, and so have shamed them out of the world.

4. I have one other consideration to present against the use of Tobacco, and that is, its tendency to create or confirm a love for alcoholic drinks. This topic is deeply interesting to all the friends of Temperance; and it may, in the end, be found more important than any other consideration I have named.

The nature of Tobacco, and the manner of its operation on the human system, should long ago have taught the world that it would kindle up a love for alcohol; and that when a love for alcohol is coupled with the use of Tobacco, a man is doubly insured as a drunkard for life. But facts are far better than abstract reasoning; and the experience of many who have abandoned Tobacco has taught us, that the cud and the pipe first led to the bottle; and that when the former was forsaken, the latter was no longer desired. It is one of the propitious signs of the times, that many friends of Temperance are waking up to this connection, and learning that they have something more to do than merely to banish the use of alcohol. Rev. Mr. Trask, of Massachusetts, who had been lecturing two years on the subject of Tobacco, says: "Tobacco and alcohol live in endearing friendship in each other's bosom. If ever Satan had twin sons, here they are." According to his observation, Tobacco and rum go hand in hand in effecting the drunkard's ruin. He adds: "It is to be feared that laws, however stringent, against in temperance, will, by-and-by, prove little better than cobwebs, unless this terrible Tobacco *mania* with the young is put back in its destructive march."

No man has a better claim to be heard on this point than Mr. Delavan, of New York. In 1845, he wrote: "I have had my fears for the safety of the Temperance cause, through the insidious influence of Tobacco. There can be no doubt but that this vile weed originates many diseases, causes premature death, and much intemperance. It is my conviction, that, while the use of Tobacco continues, intemperance will continue to curse the world. The use of Tobacco leads to the use of intoxicating drinks. They are all of one family." In 1852, he wrote: "If the habitual use of such an article as Tobacco is not sin *per se*, it would seem that ignorance of its destructive tendencies alone prevents its being so. For, unless this almost universal use of Tobacco is checked, much, if not all, that has been gained to the world by the Temperance Reformation will, I fear, be ultimately lost. Let the rising generation of lads become Tobacco-consumers, and it requires no prophetic foresight to discover that they will become consumers of strong drink also. There is an evident, if not a uniform connection between rum and Tobacco. There may have been inebriates who have not been Tobacco-consumers; but if there have been, they have not been of my acquaintance."

VI. THE CURE.

As to the method of curing the evil in question, it may be remarked, that Tobacco-using has found a place in every civilized and every savage nation on the globe. It has become implicated deeply in the agriculture and commerce of the world, so that it is a giant evil, a mighty, spreading, overwhelming flood, not to be controlled or turned back, except by united, radical, and persevering efforts. Tobacco has spread over the world, through the potency of appetite and interest. The idea which has helped its rapid spread has been, that using it was a harmless habit, or, at most, that a little would do no hurt. This idea has probably occupied the minds of the masses in all lands, and, therefore, no substantial barrier has been erected against this overflowing evil. The pulpit, the press, and even parental influence have been silent; and Temperance Societies have not wished to involve themselves in what seemed to be foreign matters.

Nothing can be done to stay the progress of this evil, unless the idea that Tobacco-using is a harmless habit can be effectually broken up. Towards this object much has already been done. Physicians of the highest eminence, and others, have shown to the world the energetic poisonous qualities of Tobacco; and that such an article could never be used habitually, without detriment to the human constitution. They have fortified their arguments with facts which even Tobacco-lovers will not be able to gainsay. Later observations, too, have shown the power of Tobacco in creating intemperate habits, and thus linked its opposers more closely with the Temperance cause than

formerly. Hereafter, we may presume that the anti-Tobacco flag will
be nailed to the Temperance mast, and that both causes will rise or fall
together.

But all this only lays the foundation for reformation, which must be carried forward by the united efforts of all the friends of humanity. Old Tobacco-
consumers should be encouraged to break off the injurious habit, with the
assurance that a little perseverance will banish the longing, tormenting appetite ; and what greater encouragement can they ask, than the testimony of
many physicians, that they have known of none who have abandoned Tobacco
who have not done it with decided advantage to their health. The experi-
ences of reformed chewers and smokers should be published to the world.
They will be demonstrations against Tobacco, "known and read of all men."

Still the habit of using Tobacco is one of dreadful power ; and we may not
always succeed with the old. A greater hope may lie in preventing the
young from entering these fearful lists. Parents should be awake, should
warn and guard their children. Christian parents will rarely fail of success.
Teachers should abstain themselves, and exert a good influence over the
young placed under their care. The pulpit and the press should break their
silence, and exhibit the evils of Tobacco as they are. But with all these
agencies, how can the plague be stayed, when the churches of Christ are so
deeply implicated as they now are in the evil ? Professing Christians sanc-
tion, by their example, the absurd and ruinous fashion, which is drawing the
young, by thousands, into this filthy vortex. And cannot the churches be
purified from a practice so unreasonable as this ? Those who now profess
religion in the Sandwich Islands were once all ardent lovers of Tobacco.
But most of the churches in these islands are pledged to be Anti-Tobacco Soci
ties. Many of the schools are pledged never to use Tobacco. Such societies
might be formed extensively among the people of every enlightened land.
And thus truth would lift up her head, and an influence go forth against the
weed, before which we might hope that, in time, the potent spell of appetite
and fashion would be dissipated, and that this abominable and filthy kind of
slavery would come to an end.

Lahaina, Sandwich Islands.

A LIST OF WORKS

By Fowlers and Wells, Clinton Hall, 131 Nassau Street, New York.

In order to accommodate "The People," residing in all parts of the United States, the under-signed Publishers will forward by return of the First Mail, any book named in the following List. The postage will be pre-paid by them, at the New York Office. By this arrangement of pre-paying postage in advance, fifty per cent. is saved to the purchaser. The price of each work, including postage, is given, so that the exact amount may be remitted. All letters containing orders, should be post-paid, and directed as follows. FOWLERS AND WELLS, Clinton Hall, 131 Nassau Street, New York.

On Phrenology.

Combe's Lectures on Phrenol-
ogy. A complete course. Bound in Muslin, $1 25.

Chart, for Recording various
velopments. Designed for Phrenologists. 6 cents.

Constitution of Man. By Geo.
Combe. Authorized Edition. Paper, 62 cts. Muslin, 87 cts.

Constitution of Man. School
Edition. Arranged with Questions. 30 cents.

Defence of Phrenology, with
Arguments and Testimony. By Dr. Boardman. Paper, 62 cents. Muslin, 87 cents.

Domestic Life, Thoughts on.
Its Concord and Discord. By N. Sizer. 15 cents.

Education Complete. Em-
bracing Physiology, Animal and Mental, Self-Culture, and Memory. In 1 vol. By O. S. Fowler. $2 50.

Education, Founded on the
Nature of Man. Dr. Spurzheim. 62 cts. Muslin, 87 cts.

Familiar Lessons on Phrenol-
ogy and Physiology. Muslin, in one volume. $1 25.

Love and Parentage : applied
to the Improvement of Offspring. 30 cents.
The same. in Muslin, including Amativeness. 75 cents.

Marriage : Its History and
Philosophy. with Directions for Happy Marriages. Bound in Paper, 50 cents. Muslin 75 cents.

Memory and Intellectual Im-
prove ent: Applied to Self-Education. By O. S. Fowler. Paper, 62 cents. Muslin, 87 cents.

Mental Science, Lectures on,
According to the Philosophy of Phrenology. By Rev. G. S. Weaver. Paper, 62 cents. Muslin, 87 cents.

Matrimony : or, Phrenology
and Physiology applied to the Selection of Congenial Companions for Life. 30 cents.

Moral and Intellectual Sci-
ence. By Combe, Gregory, and others. Muslin, $2 30.

Phrenology Proved, Illustra-
ted, and Applied. Thirty-seventh edition. A standard work on the science. Muslin, $1 25.

Phrenological Journal, Ameri-
can Monthly. Quarto, Illustrated. A year, One Dollar.

Popular Phrenology, with
Phrenological Developments. 30 cents.

Phrenology and the Scrip-
tures. By Rev. John Pierpont. 12 cents.

Phrenological Guide : Design-
ed for the Use of Students. 15 cents.

Phrenological Almanac : Illus-
trated with numerous engravings. 6 cents.

Phrenological Bust : designed
especially for Learners, showing the exact location of all the Organs of the Brain fully developed. Price, includ-ing box for packing, $1 25. [Not mailable.]

Religion, Natural and Reveal-
ed, Or the Natural Theology and Moral Bearings of Phrenology. Paper, 62 cents. Muslin, 87 cents.

Self-Culture and Perfection of
Character. Paper, 62 cents. Muslin, 87 cents.

Self-Instructor in Phrenology
and Physiology, Illustrated, with One hundred Engrav-ings. Paper, 30 cents. Muslin, 50 cents.

Synopsis of Phrenology and
Physiology. By L. N. Fowler. 15 cents.

Symbolical Head and Phreno-
logical Chart, in Map Form, showing the Natural Lan-guage of the Phrenological Organs. 25 cents.

Temperance and Tight-Lac-
ing. On the Laws of Life. By O. S. F. 15 cents.

Works of Gall, Combe, Spurz-
heim and Others, together with all works on Phrenology, for sale, wholesale and retail. Agents and Booksellers supplied, by Fowlers and Wells, New York.

Hydropathy, or Water-Cure.

"IF THE PEOPLE can be thoroughly indoctrinated in the general principles of HYDROPATHY, they will not er much, certainly not fatally, in their home application of the WATER-CURE APPLIANCES to the common disease of tae day. If they can go a step further, and make themselves acquainted with the LAWS OF LIFE AND HEALTH, they will well nigh emancipate themselves from all need of doctors of any sort."—DR. TRALL, IN HYDROPATHY FOR THE PEOPLE.

Accidents and Emergencies.
By Alfred Smee. Notes by Trall. Illustrated. 15 cents.

Bulwer, Forbes and Houghton
on the Water Treatment. One large volume. $1 25.

Cook - Book, Hydropathic.
With new Recipes. By R. T. Trall, M. D. Paper, 62 cents. Muslin, 87 cents.

Children ; Their Hydropathic
Management in Health and Disease. By Dr. Shew. $1 25.

Consumption : Its Causes, Pre-
vention and Cure. Paper, 62 cents. Muslin, 87 cents.

Curiosities of Common Water.
A Medical work. From London edition. 30 cents.

Cholera : Its Causes, Preven-
tion and Cure : and all other Bowel Complaints. 30 cts.

Confessions and Observations
of a Water Patient. By Sir E. Lytton Bulwer. 15 cts.

Errors of Physicians and Oth-
ers, in the Application of the Water-Cure. 30 cents.

Experience in Water-Cure, in
Acute and other Diseases. By Mrs. Nichols. 30 cents.

Hydropathic Encyclopedia. A
Complete System of Hydropathy and Hygiene. Illustrated. By R. T. Trall, M. D. Two volumes, with nearly One Thousand pages. Illustrated. Price, $3 00.

Hydropathy for the People.
Notes, by Dr. Trall. Paper, 62 cents. Muslin, 87 cents.

Hydropathy, or Water-Cure.
Principles, and Modes of Treatment. Dr. Shew. $1 25.

Home Treatment for Sexual
Abuses, with Hydropathic Management. A Practical Treatise for Both Sexes. By Dr. Trall. 30 cents.

Hygiene and Hydropathy,
Lectures on. By R. S. Houghton, M. D. 30 cents.

Introduction to the Water-
Cure. With First Principles. 15 cents.

Midwifery and the Diseases of
Women. A practical work. By Dr. Shew. $1 25.

Milk Trade in New York and
Vicin.ty. By Mullaly. Introduction by Trall. 30 cents.

Parent's Guide and Childbirth
Made Easy. By Mrs. H Pendleton. 60 cents.

Philosophy of Water-Cure. By
John Balbirnie, M. D. A work for beginners. 30 cts.

Pregnancy and Childbirth,
Water-Cure for Women, with cases. 30 cents.

Principles of Hydropathy ;
Invalid's Guide to Health. By D. A. Harsha. 15 cents.

Practice of Water-Cure. By
Drs. Wilson and Gully. A handy, popular work. 30 cts.

Science of Swimming : Giv-
ing Practical Instruction to Learners. 12 cents.

Water-Cure Library ; Em-
bracing the Most Important Works on the Subject. In seven large 12mo. volumes. A Family work. $6 00.

Water-Cure in America, con-
taining Reports of Three Hundred Cases. $1 25.

Water and Vegetable Diet in
Scrofula, Cancer, Asthma, &c. By Dr. Lamb. Notes by Shew. 62 cents. Muslin, 87 cents.

Water-Cure in Every Known
Disease. By J. H. Rausse. 62 cents. Muslin, 87 cents.

Water-Cure Manual ; A Pop-
ular Work on Hydropathy. 62 cents. Muslin, 87 cents.

Water-Cure Almanac, Con-
taining much important matter for all classes. 6 cents.

Water-Cure Journal and Her-
ald of Reforms. Devoted to Hydropathy and Medical Reform. Published monthly, at One Dollar a Year.

FOWLERS AND WELLS have all works on PHYSIOLOGY, HYDROPATHY, and the Natural Sciences generally. Booksellers supplied on the most liberal terms. AGENTS wanted in every state, county, and town. These works are universally popular, and thousands might be sold where they have never yet been introduced.

TO PREVENT MISCARRIAGES, DELAYS OR OMISSIONS, all letters and other communications should, in ALL CASES, be post-paid, and directed to the Publishers, as follows :—FOWLERS AND WELLS, Clinton Hall, 131 Nassau St., New York.

THE PUBLISHERS would respectfully refer strangers, Agents, and Country dealers, to any of the principal Publishers in New York, Philadelphia, Boston, or other cities, for evidence of their ability to fulfil all contracts, and to meet all engagements. They have been many years before the public, engaged in the publishing business in the City of New York.

Physiology, Mesmerism and Psychology.

ON PHYSIOLOGY.

Amativeness ; or, Evils and
Remedies of Excessive and Perverted Sexuality, with Advice to the Married and Single. 15 cents.

Combe on Infancy ; or, the
Physiological and Moral Management of Children. Illustrated. Paper, 62 cents. Muslin, 87 cents.

Combe's Physiology, Applied
to the Improvement of Mental and Physical Education. Notes by Fowler. Paper, 62 cents. Muslin, 87 cents.

Chronic Diseases, Especially
Nervous Diseases of Women. Important work. 30 cents.

Digestion, Physiology of. The
Principles of Dietetics. By Andrew Combe. 30 cents.

Food and Diet: Containing an
Analysis of every kind of Food and Drink. By Pereira. Paper, 87 cents. Muslin, $1 25.

Generation, Philosophy of :
Its Abuses, Causes, Prevention, and Cure. 30 cents.

Hereditary Descent: Its Laws
and Facts applied to Human Improvement. O. S. F. New edition. Paper, 62 cents. Muslin, 87 cents.

Maternity : Or the Bearing
and Nursing of Children, including Female Education. O. S. Fowler. Paper, 62 cents. Muslin, 87 cents.

Natural Laws of Man. By Dr.
Spurzheim. A good work. 30 cents.

Natural History of Man. By
Dr Newman. Illustrated. Paper, 62 cts. Muslin, 87 cts.

Physiology, Animal and Mental: Applied to Health of Body and Power of Mind.
By O. S. F. Paper, 62 cents Muslin, 87 cents.

Reproductive Organs; Their
Diseases, Causes, and Cure Hydropathically. 15 cents.

Sober and Temperate Life :
with Notes and Illustrations by Louis Cornaro. 30 cents.

Tobacco : Its Effect on th
Body and Mind. By Dr. Shew. 30 cents.

Teeth : Their Structure, Dis
ease, and Management, with many Engravings. 15

Tea and Coffee : Their Physical, Intellectual and Moral Effects.
By Alcott. 15 cts.

Tobacco, Use of; Its Physical,
Intellectual and Moral Effects. By Alcott. 15 cents.

Vegetable Diet, as Sanctioned
by Medical Men, and Experience in all ages. By Dr. Alcott. Paper, 62 cents. Muslin, 87 cents.

MESMERISM AND PSYCHOLOGY.

Biology ; Or the Principles of
the Human Mind. By Alfred Smee. Illustrated. 30 cts.

Electrical Psychology, Philosophy of, in Twelve Lectures.
By Dr. J. B. Dods. Paper, 62 cents. Muslin, 87 cents.

Elements of Animal Magnetism ; Or Process and Practical Application.
15 cents.

Fascination, or the Philosophy
of Charming (Magnetism). Illustrating the Principles of Life. Paper, 50 cents. Muslin, 87 cents.

Mental Alchemy. A Treatise
on the Mind and Nervous System. By Williams. 62 cts.

Macrocosm and Microcosm ; or
the Universe Without and the Universe Within. By Fishbough. Scientific Work. Paper, 62 cts. Muslin, 87 cents.

Philosophy of Mesmerism and
Clairvoyance, Six Lectures, with Instruction. 30 cents.

Psychology, or the Science of
the Soul. By Haddock. Illustrated. 30 cents

Spiritual Intercourse, Philosophy of, an Explanation of Modern Mysteries.
62 cents

Supernal Theology, and Life
in the Spheres. By Owen G. Warren. 30 cents

EITHER OF THESE WORKS may be ordered and received by return of the FIRST MAIL, postage prepaid by the Publishers. Please address all letters, post-paid, to   FOWLERS AND WELLS,
Clinton Hall, 131 Nassau Street, New York.

N. B. Please be particular to give us the name of your POST OFFICE, COUNTY and STATE.

Phonography and Miscellaneous.

When single copies of these works are wanted, the amount, in postage stamps, small change, or bank notes may be enclosed in a letter and sent to the Publishers, who will forward the books by return of the FIRST MAIL.

ON PHONOGRAPHY.

Constitution of the United
States, in Phonography, Corresponding style. 15 cents.

Declaration of Independence,
in Phonography, a sheet; for framing. 15 cents.

Phonographic Teacher; Being
an Inductive Exposition of Phonography, intended for a school book, and to afford complete instruction to those who have not the assistance of an oral teacher. By E. Webster. In Boards. 45 cents.

Phonographic Envelopes,
Large and Small, containing Brief Explanations of Phonography and its Utility. Price, per thousand, $3 25.

Phonographic Alphabet, upon
Enamelled Card. Price, per hundred, $3 00.

Phonographic Word-Signs, on
Card. Per hundred copies, $3 00.

The Universal Phonographer :
Monthly Journal, devoted to the Dissemination of Phonography, and to Verbatim Reporting, with Practical Instruction to Learners, Printed in Phonography. [No discount on this work.] Price, A YEAR, $1 00.

MISCELLANEOUS.

Botany for all Classes ; Con-
taining a Floral Dictionary, with numerous Illustrations. Paper, 62 cents. Muslin, 87 cents.

Chemistry, Applied to Physi-
ology, Agriculture, and Commerce. By Liebig. 25 cts.

Delia's Doctors ; or, A Glance
Behind the Scenes. By Miss Hanna Gardner Creamer. Paper, 62 cents. Muslin, 87 cents.

Essay on Wages, Showing the
Necessity of a Workingman's Tariff. 15 cents.

Familiar Lessons on Astrono-
my. Designed for Children and Youth in Schools and Families. Mrs. Fowler. Paper, 62 cts. Muslin, 87 cts.

Future of Nations, A Lecture.
By Louis Kossuth. Revised by the author. 12 cents.

Hints toward Reforms, in Lec-
tures, Addresses, and other Writings. By H. Greeley. Second Edition, Enlarged, with Crystal Palace. $1 25.

Hopes and Helps for the Young
of Both Sexes. By Rev. G. S. Weaver. An excellent work. Paper, 62 cents. Muslin, 87 cents.

Human Rights, and their Po-
litical Guaranties. By Judge Hurlbut. An important work. Paper, 62 cents. Muslin, 87 cents.

Home for All : New, Cheap,
Convenient, and Superior Mode of Building. 87 cents.

Immortality Triumphant.
The Existence of a God, with the Evidence. By Rev. J. B. Dods. Paper, 62 cents. Muslin, 87 cents.

Innovation Entitled to a Full
and Candid Hearing. By John Patterson. 15 cents.

Literature and Art. By S
Margaret Fuller. Introduction by Horace Greeley. $1 25

Labor : Its History and Pros-
pects. Use and Abuse of Wealth. By Owen. 30 cents

Power of Kindness ; Inculca-
ting the Christian Principles of Love over Physical Force. Paper, 30 cents. Muslin, 50 cents.

Population, Theory of. The
Law of Animal Fertility. Introduction by Trall. 15 cts.

Temperance Reformation—
Its History from the First Temperance Society to the Adoption of the Maine Law. By Armstrong. $1 25.

The Student : A Monthly Mag-
azine, Devoted to the Physical, Moral, and Intellectual Improvement of Youth. Amply Illustrated. Price, One Dollar a Year.

Woman : Her Education and
Influence. With an Introduction by Mrs. C. M. Kirkland. Paper, 50 cents. Muslin, 87 cents.

Woman, in all Ages and Na-
tions. An Authentic History, from the Earliest Ages. Paper, 62 cents. Muslin, 87 cents.

THESE works may be ordered in large or small quantities. A liberal discount will be made to AGENTS, and others, who buy to sell again. They may be sent by Express or as Freight, by Railroad, Steamships, Sailing Vessels, by Stage or Canal, to any City, Town, or Village in the United States, the Canadas, to Europe, or any place on the Globe.

Checks or drafts, for large amounts, on New York, Philadelphia, or Boston, always preferred. We pay cost of exchange

☞ All letters should be post-paid, and addressed as follows :—

FOWLERS AND WELLS,
[Name the Post Office, Co., and State.]
Clinton Hall, 131 Nassau St., New York.

Our Illustrated Journals.

FOWLERS AND WELLS publish the following PERIODICALS. They have an aggregate circulation of about ONE HUNDRED THOUSAND COPIES. These Popular and Professional SERIALS afford an excellent opportunity for bringing before the Public with Pictorial Illustrations all subjects of interest, Physiological, Educational, Agricultural, Mechanical, and Commercial.

THE WATER-CURE JOURNAL, AND HERALD OF REFORMS. Devoted to Hydropathy, its Philosophy and Practice, to Physiology and Anatomy, with illustrative engravings, to Dietetics, Exercise, Clothing, Occupations, Amusements, and those Laws which govern Life and Health. Published Monthly, in convenient form for binding, at One Dollar a Year in advance.

The Water-Cure Journal holds a high rank in the science of health; always, ready straightforward, and plain-spoken, it unfolds the law of our physical nature, without any pretensions to the technicalities of science, but in a form as attractive and refreshing as the sparkling element of which it treats. We know of no American periodical which presents a greater abundance of valuable information on all subjects relating to human progress and welfare.—[New-York Tribune.

This is, unquestionably, the most popular Health Journal in the world.—[New-York Daily Evening Post.

Every man, woman, and child who loves health; who desires happiness, its direct result; who wants to "live while he does live," "live till he dies," and really live, instead of being a mere walking corpse, should become at once a reader of this Journal, and practise its precepts.—[Fountain Journal.

THE AMERICAN PHRENOLOGICAL JOURNAL. A Repository of Science, Literature, and General Intelligence; Devoted to Phrenology, Physiology, Education, Magnetism, Psychology, Mechanism, Agriculture, Horticulture, Architecture, the Arts and Sciences, and to all those Progressive Measures which are calculated to Reform, Elevate, and Improve Mankind. Illustrated with numerous portraits and other engravings. A beautiful Quarto, suitable for binding. Published Monthly, at one Dollar a Year in advance.

This is the only work of the kind in the country; indeed, the editors, from their intimate and profound knowledge of the science of Phrenology, are the only persons who could make up a work of such varied and singular excellence. It may be termed the standard authority in all matters pertaining to Phrenology, while the beautiful typography of the Journal, and the superior character of the numerous illustrations, are not exceeded in any work with which we are acquainted.—[Model American Courier, Philadelphia.

A Journal containing such a mass of interesting matter, devoted to the highest happiness and interests of men, written in the clear and lively style of its practised editors, and afforded at the "ridiculously low price" of one dollar a year, must succeed in running up its present large circulation [50,000 copies !] to a much higher figure.—[New York Tribune.

THE ILLUSTRATED HYDROPATHIC QUARTERLY REVIEW. A New Professional Magazine, devoted to Medical Reform, embracing articles by the best writers, on Anatomy, Physiology, Pathology, Surgery, Therapeutics, Midwifery, etc., Reports of Remarkable Cases in General Practice, Criticisms on the Theory and Practice of the various Opposing Systems of Medical Science, Reviews of New Publications of all Schools of Medicine, Reports of the Progress of Health Reform in all its Aspects, etc., etc., with appropriate illustrations. Each number contains from 190 to 200 octavo pages, at Two Dollars a Year.

In addition to the widely circulated monthly journals issued by these enterprising publishers, we have the New Hydropathic Quarterly Review, a professional repository of facts and experiments in medical science, as well as of critical judgments on different modes of practice, examined in the light of hydropathic principles; edited by the most distinguished members of that school. It is filled with articles of permanent value, which ought to be read by every American.—[New York Tribune.

COMMUNICATIONS, NEW BOOKS for notice or review, ADVERTISEMENTS, and SUBSCRIPTIONS, should be addressed to the PUBLISHERS,

FOWLERS AND WELLS,

Boston, 142 Washington Street. }
Philadelphia, 231 Arch Street. }

CLINTON HALL, 131 Nassau Street, New-York.